PALEO KID SNACKS:

27 Super Easy Recipes
That Kids Can't Get Enough Of
(Primal Gluten Free Kids Cookbook)

Kate Evans Scott

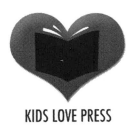

KIDS LOVE PRESS

This book is dedicated to my two beautiful children.

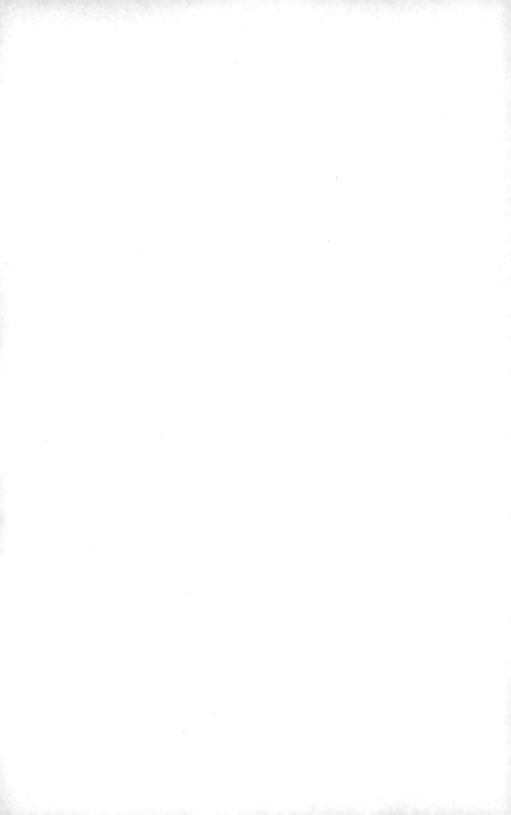

TABLE OF CONTENTS

SAUCES

SAVORY SNACKS

DAIRY-FREE MILKS

ACKNOWLEDGMENTS

Thank You to my friends and family once again for your encouragement. Your support has truly helped make this book a reality.

It's a wonderful feeling to know that this book is finding its way into the hands of other like-minded Paleo lovers. This book is for you!

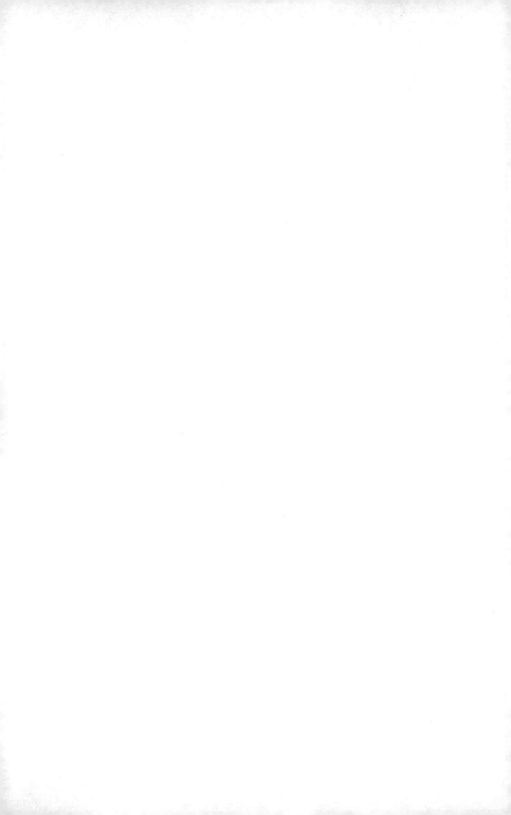

PALEO KIDS SNACK-ATTACK

Kids love to snack, and there's a good reason for it. They need the energy to fuel their rapidly growing bodies. With stomachs that aren't large enough to accommodate the necessary amount of food to carry them from meal to meal, they need to grab healthy snacks in between. Unfortunately, the food industry has latched onto the "snack" and turned it into a naughty word. Indeed, the kind of snacking promoted by the large munchies-food corporations is not healthy at all. Cheese crackers, bear shaped cookies, twisted pretzels and pudding cups do not provide the kind of nutrition necessary for healthy development. These kinds of snacks can cause rapid insulin fluctuations (sugar rushes and subsequent crashes), inflammation, behavior issues, weight gain, and mood swings. They provide almost no nutritional value, and do more to hinder than to aid in the child's work of maturing into healthy young adults.

As Paleo parents, you've already made the choice to cut out the junk and return instead to the wholesome diet that our bodies were designed to consume. While the meals you provide your children are likely already packed with protein, fiber and vital nutrients, your kids will still need to eat in between. Remember, their bellies are too small to hold everything they need at once! So, you've planned your breakfasts, lunches, and dinners, and now you have to worry about snacks too? No! You don't have to worry at all!

UH-OH, PALEO! WHAT IS THIS DIET?
(THE PALEO KID EXCERPT)

Starting on the paleo diet is like taking a step back in time... way back in time... It's a gastro-adventure that takes you backward two million years to the paleolithic era, when humans were a hunter-gatherer society. That means that people lived on wild game and the plants, fruits, and nuts they gathered from their environment.

When human beings started cultivating grains and raising animals for meat and dairy 10,000 years ago, we began suffering from chronic illnesses like heart disease, type 2 diabetes, obesity, depression, memory loss, and other inflammatory diseases. Tribal people living today that eat similar diets to our paleolithic ancestors do not suffer from these life-threatening diseases. We have to assume that it has to do with their diet and lifestyle.

If you do the paleo diet right, you won't feel hungry and crave the foods you've eliminated. Instead, you'll feel satiated, vibrant, and healthy!

WHAT KIND OF SNACKS DO MY KIDS NEED?

Snacks can be as simple as a piece of fresh fruit or a savory plate of bacon-wrapped chicken nuggets. With a few basic sauces prepared ahead and kept in the refrigerator, you can have quick bites at your child's fingertips. In fact, some of these snacks could be served as appetizers at dinner parties, arranged in a bento box for a Paleo lunch, or paired with a meat or veggie dish for a nice weekday dinner. A snack doesn't necessarily have to crunch, gush, or come in a small colorful bag! A snack is simply anything you eat between meals.

The most important quality of your child's snack is that it helps fulfill his or her nutrition requirements. If you noticed that your son usually just eats fruit salad for breakfast, make sure he has a protein snack- like chicken cubes with barbecue sauce- sometime midmorning, or you might see his energy waning. If your daughter prefers poached eggs with bacon and avocado for breakfast, set out a tray of fresh veggies and ranch dip for pre-lunch noshing. The same goes for the afternoon snack. In this way, you will use these mini-meals to balance out your children's daily nutritional intake.

WHAT ABOUT THEIR TEETH?

Has your dentist scared you off of snacks because of their potential to cause tooth decay? If you are concerned about the impact of snacking on your child's teeth, just make sure they brush after they eat. You can also reduce the risk for tooth decay by steering clear of chewy, sugary, dried fruits and instead opt for fresh veggies and meats between meals.

Evidence also shows that the use of xylitol products helps strengthen enamel and reduce the risk of tooth decay. Xylitol is naturally derived from tree bark and is a great sweetener. You can often find it in the form of gum, mints, mouthwash, sugar substitute, and toothpaste at your local health food store. Just be careful to check the label, as some xylitol is now being manufactured from corn. It still has the same positive effects, but if you're steering clear of grains then you'll want the original bark-based xylitol.

TRICKS OF THE TRADE

Some children are just way too busy to stop and eat. That block tower isn't going to build itself, you know! It's no good to force feed your over-involved child. But if you are seeing them crash and burn because their stores of energy get completely depleted before they refuel, then you'll want to slip in a snack. The best trick for the busy child is to set out a plate of food where they can see it and graze. If your little construction worker drives his dump truck past the coffee table and snags an almond cracker topped with apple butter, the nutrition is in! Mission accomplished.

Other children are painfully picky. The grazing method is also good for the picky eaters, but I have another trick to tuck up your sleeve for those times when you just know your child will love something, but you just can't get them to try it... We'll call it the "my snack" trick. Let's say that you really want your picky daughter to try a turkey-pesto rollup. Instead of sitting her down with a plate and telling her to eat, quietly make the dish and sit down with it yourself. Relax, grab a cup of tea, and enjoy your delicious snack. Soon enough, you are sure to have your daughter up on your lap asking what you're eating.

Say, "Oh, it's a rollup." Take a bite and look like you really enjoy it, but don't push it on her. When she asks if she can have a bite say, "Hmmm... I'm not sure." Before you know it, she will be begging for one! If she tries it and doesn't like it, be patient. I takes about three times tasting a new food before a child will become accustom to the flavor.

HEALTHY SNACKING: FOOD FOR THOUGHT, FOOD FOR LIFE

Bottom line is that kids need snacks, and those snacks need to be healthy. Your children rely on you to help them form their relationship to food. Their eating patterns now as young children have a huge impact on their food choices and their eating behaviors well into adulthood. By providing them with healthy Paleo meals and nutritious snacks, you are giving them a solid foundation for a lifetime of wellness.

BASIC FOOD LIST

Here is a food guideline to get you started. Remember, there is a little bit of wiggle room, as even the Paleo diet experts disagree about certain foods. If you are unsure, you should always do your own research and tailor your diet to your specific needs.

Vegetables and Sea Vegetables: You can eat any and all vegetables. In fact, you should eat a "rainbow" of vegetables, from red to violet, in order to give your body a wide variety of vitamins and nutrients. Sea veggies, like seaweed and algae, are especially good for you.

Fruits: Eat all the fruits. These can be fresh, cooked, or dried. However, if you're trying to lose weight or if you have a problem with tooth decay, you may want to limit dried fruits.

Meats, Fish & Eggs: You will eat a lot of meat and eggs on the Paleo diet, as did our hunter-gatherer ancestors. Protein plays a huge role in proper brain and muscle development, and since you're not going to eat any legumes or grains, meat and eggs become an even more important source of this vital building block.

It is always best to eat meat and eggs that came from pasture raised animals that were fed a diet similar to what they would eat in the wild. Always stay away from meats that have added preservatives or flavor enhancers, like nitrites or MSG. All different fish species are healthy choices, just be conscious of high mercury levels and choose fish with ecologically friendly harvesting practices. Here are some options: Turkey, chicken, goat, lamb, pork, organ meat (liver, gizzards, heart), game meats (pheasant, duck, deer, bison, goose, quail), beef, eggs (from chicken, duck, emu, etc), fish, shell fish, and fish eggs.

Nuts, Seeds, and Butters: All nuts and seeds are good, as well as the butters made from them. Keep in mind that peanuts are NOT nuts. They are legumes, and thus are NOT part of the Paleo diet. Almond butter makes a great replacement for peanut butter, and there are many mild nut butters that work well in baking.

Fats and Oils: Use fats and oils sparingly. Remember that you can not use grain oils, like corn oil or peanut oil. But there are a lot of great substitutes: lard, tallow, bacon grease, olive oil, coconut oil, walnut oil, avocado oil, hazelnut oil, flaxseed oil (unheated).

Drinks: Filtered or spring water should be your main drink. You can also add herbal tea, coconut water, and freshly juiced fruits and vegetables. Stay away from soda, bottled juice and juice drinks.

Seasoning: Most spices are fine, including sea salt (NOT refined iodized salt).

The following foods/beverages are okay in moderation, but you don't want to overdo them: Coffee, chocolate, caffeinated tea, raw honey, stevia, agave, grade B maple syrup.

FOODS TO AVOID

This is going to be a tough transition for some children, as they are going to have to give up some foods that they love, like cheese, pasta, and bread. But once you start cooking some of the delicious recipes in this book, they will get used to a new, healthier way of eating. They'll start to feel good, and they will stop missing the pizza and sodas!

Cereal Grains: Wheat, rice, barley, corn millet, spelt, kamut, rice, amaranth, sorghum, rye, oats, quinoa, or anything made out of grains (flour, noodles, bread, crackers).

Legumes: All beans are out of the picture, including soybeans (tofu, too) and peanuts. Eliminate black beans, pintos, lentils, peas, lima beans, black-eyed peas, garbanzo beans (hummus), kidney beans, etc.

Sugar and Artificial Sweeteners: white sugar, brown sugar, turbinado sugar, refined maple syrup, high fructose corn syrup, corn syrup, molasses, refined honey, sucralose, aspartame, Splenda, Equal.

Highly Processed Oils and Most Vegetable Oils: Any oil that comes from a seed or legume is not acceptable, like soybean oil, corn oil, safflower oil, and grape seed oil. Also stay away from hydrogenated, partially hydrogenated and refined oils.

Dairy Products: This includes butter, yogurt, cheese and milk from cows, goats, sheep and buffalo. Basically, if it comes from an animal's teat, it is not allowed on the diet. However, that is up for debate in the Paleo community. Do your research. If you choose to eat some dairy, make sure that it is full-fat, raw (unpasteurized), organic and grass-fed, fermented dairy.

QUICK & DELICIOUS

Smoothies are a quick and delicious way to fill your kids with the vitamins, nutrients, and fiber necessary to keep their bodies going. You can use just about any combination of fruits, juices, and milks to create your own perfect flavor, or you can use one of the tried-and-true recipes we've provided here.

TIP: Smoothies are perfect for cleaning up the icebox of super-ripened fruits. When you notice your banana is a little brown, or your pears are slightly too soft, cut them up and store them in airtight containers in the freezer. Frozen, ripe fruit makes your smoothie cold without adding ice.

SMOOTHIES
- Tropical Smoothie -
- Green Monster Smoothie -
- Strawberry Shake -

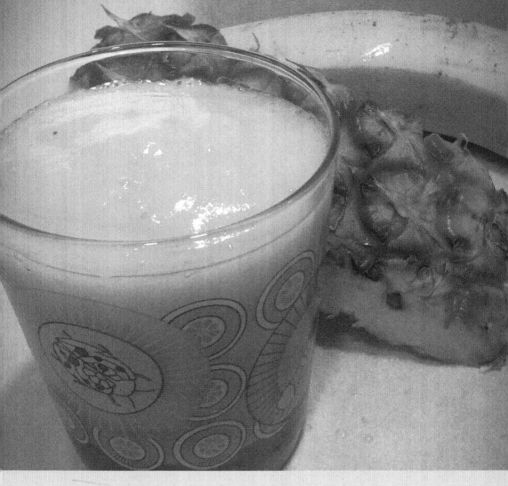

Tropical Smoothie

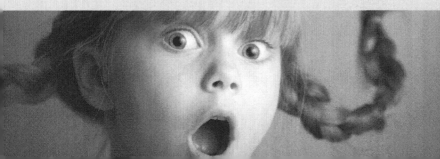

TROPICAL SMOOTHIE

Smoothies are one of the quickest, most nutritious snacks that kids absolutely love! Packed with all the nutrition of juice, the smoothie retains the fiber necessary for healthy digestion. While you can certainly mix and match your fruits any way you like, this tropical smoothie is a favorite for its consistency and light, refreshing flavor. It tastes like a drink you'd enjoy on a beach with a little umbrella!

Tropical Smoothie Recipe

Ingredients:

- 1 cup cubed frozen mango
- 1 cup fresh cubed pineapple
- 1 medium – large ripe banana, peeled and sliced
- ½ cup orange juice

Directions: Combine all ingredients in a blender or food processor. Process on high until completely smooth. Pour into two glasses and enjoy!

Serving size: 8 oz   Yields: 2 servings
Prep Time: 5 minutes   Cook time: 0
Total time: 5 minutes

YUM YUM YUMMY SNACKS!

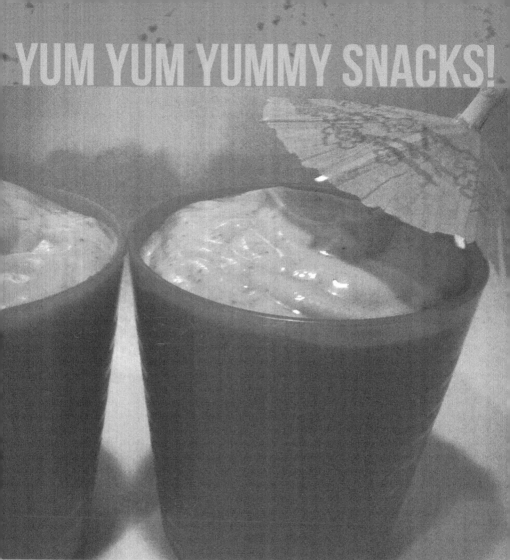

Green Monster Smoothie

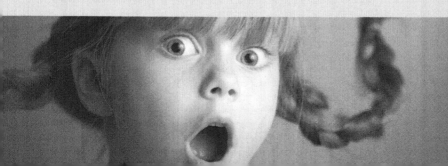

GREEN MONSTER SMOOTHIE

Packed with protein and essential amino acids, this smoothie is a delicious way to give your kids their vital nutrients. The avocado and coconut milk make this an absolutely delicious drink that has the texture of a milkshake rather than a fruit drink. For an even creamier version with added protein, freeze one cup of coconut milk in an ice cube tray ahead of time and use the coconut-cubes in place of ice. You can find the full-fat (NOT light) coconut milk in the Asian food section of most grocery stores.

Green Monster Smoothie Recipe

Ingredients:

- 1 cup spinach, loosely packed
- 1 ripe avocado
- 1 cup ice
- ½ cup coconut milk
- 1 kiwi
- 1 ripe pear
- 2 tbsp raw honey

Directions: With a sharp knife, cut avocado all the way around the center from stem to base. Twist open and remove pit. Scoop flesh into the blender and discard skin.

Rinse the pear. Using the same sharp knife, quarter the pear and remove core and seeds. Cut into chunks and add to the avocado. Peel and slice the kiwi. Add to the blender.

Add the washed baby spinach, ice, honey, and coconut milk. Blend on high until completely smooth, about 3 minutes with a regular blender. (A Vitamix or Magic Bullet will be quicker.)

Pour into two cups and enjoy!

Serving size: 8 oz   Yields: 2 servings
Prep time: 5 minutes   Blend time: 3 minutes
Total time: 8 minutes

YUM YUM YUMMY SNACKS!

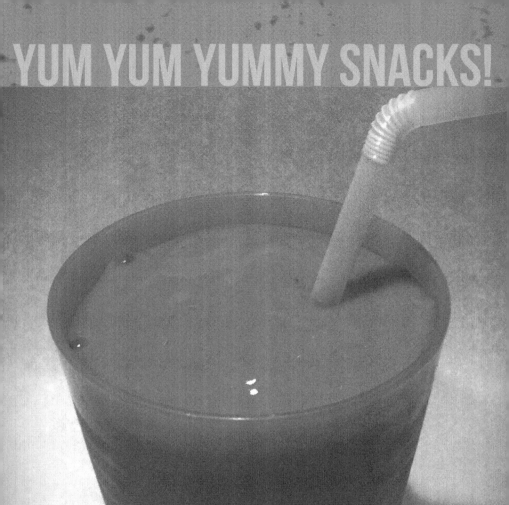

Strawberry Shake

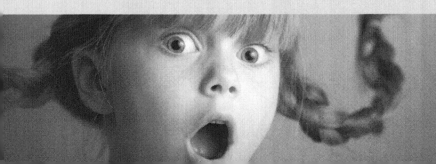

STRAWBERRY MILKSHAKE

It's a milkshake... No, it's a smoothie! The addition of vanilla and milk to the frozen strawberries and bananas gives this smoothie the flavor and mouth-feel of a creamy milkshake. My son claims that this is the best smoothie he's ever had, and I won't argue with him on that one.

Strawberry Milkshake Recipe

Ingredients:

- 1 cup frozen strawberries
- 1 large ripe banana, peeled
- 1/3 cup almond milk (can substitute coconut milk)
- 1/2 tsp vanilla extract

Directions: Place all ingredients into the blender and process on high until smooth, about three minutes. Pour into two glasses and enjoy!

Serving size: 8 ounces Yields: 2 servings
Prep time: 5 minutes Cook time: 0
Total time: 5 minutes

SLOW SWEETS

Most kids have a decent-sized sweet tooth, but they don't need candy or cookies to be satisfied. Those kinds of refined sugary snacks are contributing to a wide array of health issues affecting our youth, including diabetes and depression. However, unrefined sugars like those found in fruits and raw honey, are released slowly into the body providing a consistent source of energy throughout the day.

SWEET SNACKS
- Trail Mix -
- Grapesicles-
- Apples & Cinnamon Dip -
- Graham Crackers -
- Fruit Salad -
- Banana Bowl -
- Mango-Fruit Roller -

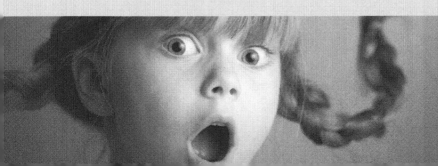

YUM YUM YUMMY SNACKS!

Trail Mix

TRAIL MIX

Trail mix is a great snack to throw in a baggie and take to the park or on a road trip. It goes well in lunch boxes and can sit out for all-day munching. Full of protein and fiber, as well as vitamins and essential fatty acids from dried coconut, you really can't lose with a handful of crunchy, chewy, trail mix. It can also be completely customized. Mix banana chips, macadamia nuts and dried mango bits together for a tropical twist. Or, maybe you'd be interested in pecans and dried apples. Anything goes!

Simple Trail Mix Recipe

Ingredients:

- ½ cup unsalted cashews
- ½ cup unsalted almonds
- ½ cup shredded or flaked, unsweetened dried coconut
- ¼ cup dried cranberries
- ¼ cup raisins

Directions: Place all ingredients in a zip-top plastic bag or a mason jar with lid. Shake until mixed well. Store right in the bag or mason jar! No fuss, no muss.

Serving size: ½ cup   Yields: 5 servings
Prep time: 5 minutes   Cook time: 0
Total time: 5 minutes

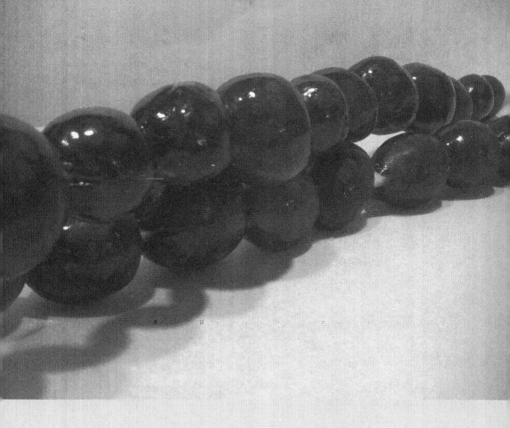

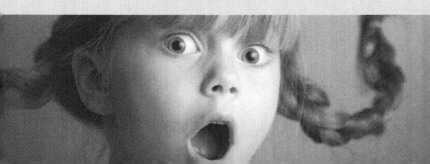

Grapesicles

GRAPESICLES

These are an absolute summer favorite! When the grapes freeze, the insides turn into tiny little bite-sized popsicles that burst with flavor. Grapes contain polyphenols, resveratrol, and saponins, which make this little treat a powerhouse for heart health. Make a big batch and keep them in a large, airtight container for hot summer afternoons.

Grapesicles Recipe

Ingredients:

* 20 seedless grapes, any color
* 2 skewers

Directions: Rinse the grapes. Poke a skewer through the stem-hole of the first grape, and push it down as far as possible onto the skewer. Repeat until the skewer is full, about ten grapes. Fill the second skewer in the same fashion.

Wrap the skewered grapes in parchment paper, paper towel, or plastic wrap and freeze for at least five hours or overnight. Keep wrapped and frozen up to one week. Serve frozen.

Serving size: 1 skewer   Yields: 2 servings
Prep time: 5 minutes   Freeze time: 5 hours – overnight
Total time: 5 hours, 5 minutes

YUM YUM YUMMY SNACKS!

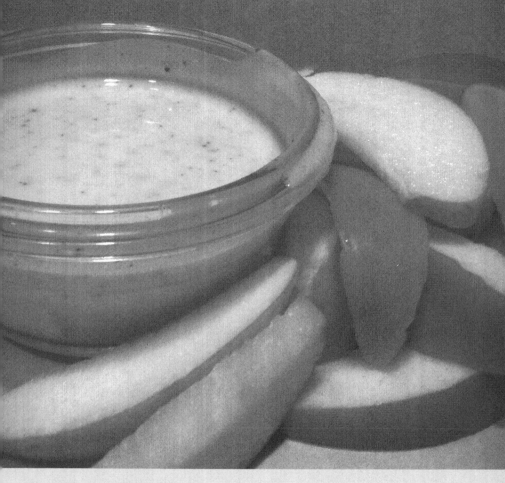

Apples & Cinnamon Dip

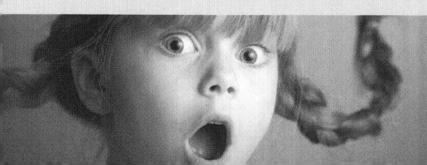

APPLES AND CINNAMON DIP

Most kids like to dip. An apple is good, but an apple dunked in creamy, sweet goodness turns an ordinary fruit into a dessert-like treat. It takes a little planning ahead to make this dip thick like the fruit dips you might find in the white tubs at the store, but you could use it right away if you're in a pinch. It will just be a little bit runny. Alternately, keep a can of full-fat coconut milk in the fridge so it's already thick when you need it.

Apples And Cinnamon Dip Recipe

Ingredients:

• 2 apples
• ½ cup coconut milk, full-fat
• 2 tbsp raw honey, softened
• ½ tsp ground cinnamon

Directions: Whisk together coconut milk, honey, and cinnamon. Cover and refrigerate at least 2 hours. This thickens the coconut milk, making this dip stick to the apples like, kind of like yogurt dip.

Before serving, wash, core, and slice two apples. Serve with the chilled cinnamon dip.

Serving size: ½ apple   Yields: 4 servings
Prep time: 5 min   Refrigeration time: 2 hours
Apple prep: 5 min   Total Time: 10 minutes

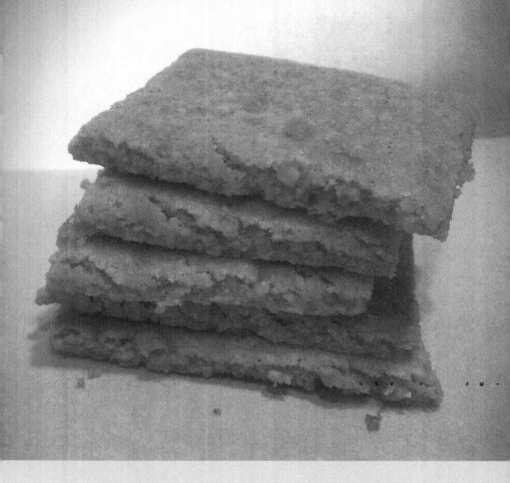

Graham Crackers

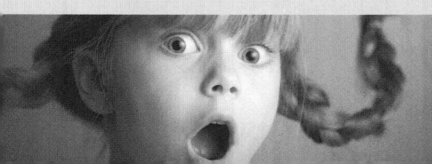

GRAHAM CRACKERS

I recently took these crackers to a play date, and just about every parent there asked me for the recipe! I had one mom tell me that she couldn't stop eating them. Make a double batch of almond graham crackers and keep them in a sealed container. I'd say that they'll keep up to a week, but they probably won't last until tomorrow!

Graham Crackers Recipe

Ingredients:

- 2 ¼ c.   Blanched almond meal (or finely ground almonds)
- 3 tbsp   Coconut oil
- 3 tbsp   Grade B maple syrup
- 1 tsp   Cinnamon
- 1 tsp   Vanilla extract
- ¼ tsp   Baking soda

Directions: Preheat oven to 325°F. Line a baking sheet with parchment paper.

Place all ingredients into a medium sized bowl. Mix with a hand mixer set on low until all ingredients are well blended and a dough ball begins to form. Remove the dough ball to the parchment-lined baking sheet.

Cover the dough ball with another sheet of parchment. With a rolling pin, roll out the dough until it is very thin, about 1/8 inch. Discard the top sheet of parchment. Prick the dough with a fork every few inches.

Bake in a preheated oven for 12 – 15 minutes, until the crackers are browned and firm to the touch. Remove from oven and cut immediately into 2-inch squares with a pizza cutter or large, sharp knife. Allow to cool in pan.

When the crackers are cooled, serve plain or topped with a dollop of apple butter! Store in an airtight container for up to 10 days.

Serving size: 3 crackers   Yields: 8 servings (24 crackers)
Prep time: 15 minutes   Cook time: 15 minutes
Total time: 30 minutes

YUM YUM YUMMY SNACKS!

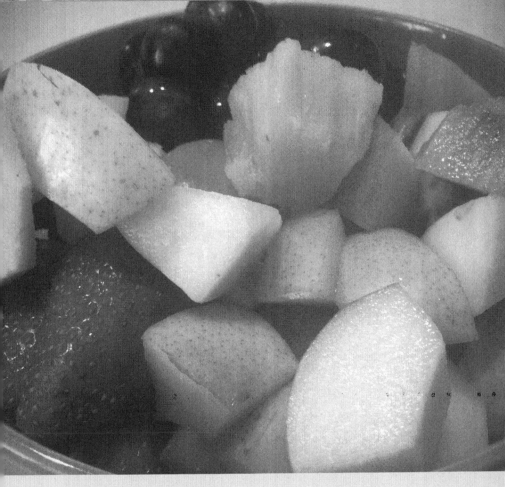

Fruit Salad

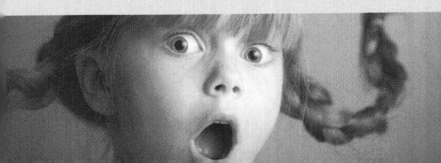

FRUIT SALAD

Kids love to make fruit salad. It's pretty. It's delicious. It's simple, and it's nutritious. Let your child (even a toddler) use a colander to rinse and a plastic knife to chop. Making a snack quickly becomes a fun and meaningful activity. Even the smallest children can create a beautiful, colorful dish to share with their friends and family.

Fruit Salad Recipe

Ingredients:

- 1 cup cubed pineapple
- 1 cup strawberries, stemmed and cut in half
- 1 ripe pear
- 1 cup grapes
- 1 kiwi
- 1 tbsp lemon juice (optional)

Directions: Wash the strawberries and grapes. Set on a towel to dry. Rinse and dry the pear. Slice it in half and remove the core and stem. Cut into bite-sized pieces and place into a large bowl.

Cut the stems off of the strawberries. Slice the larger berries in half and place in the bowl with the pears. Place washed grapes in the bowl. (For small children, cut the grapes in half.)

With a sharp paring knife, peel the skin off the kiwi. Slice into bite-sized chunks and place in bowl. Turn fruit over with a spoon to mix.

If you are going to save the fruit salad for later, sprinkle lemon juice over the top and turn to mix. This will prevent the fruit from browning.

*You can use any combination of fruits that you like! Just remember that bananas will go bad quickly, so only use them if you are eating the salad right away.

Serving size: 1 cup   Yields: 4 servings
Prep time: 10 minutes   Cook time: 0
Total time: 10 minutes

YUM YUM YUMMY SNACKS!

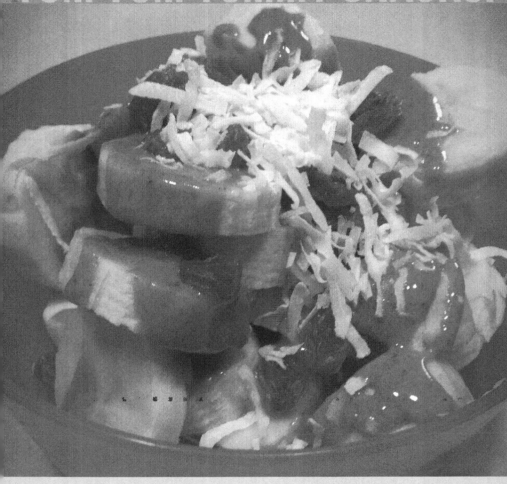

Banana Bowl

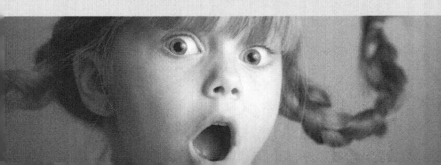

BANANA BOWL

This snack is so sweet, crunchy, and flavorful that it almost feels like dessert! Kids can prepare the banana bowl all by themselves, or you can do it for them in just a couple of minutes without even dirtying a cutting board or mixing bowl. The almond butter generally has a slightly runny consistency, so it's easy to pour like a sauce. If it seems a bit firm, just leave it on the counter or warm it in the microwave before you're ready to get started.

Banana Bowl Recipe

Ingredients:

- 1 banana
- 1 tbsp almond butter
- 1 tsp golden raisins
- 1 tsp shredded, unsweetened coconut

Directions: Peel and slice the banana into your small serving bowl. Drizzle with almond butter and top with raisins and coconut.

Serving size: About 1 cup   Yields: 1 serving
Prep time: 3 minutes   Cook time: 0
Total time: 3 minutes

YUM YUM YUMMY SNACKS!

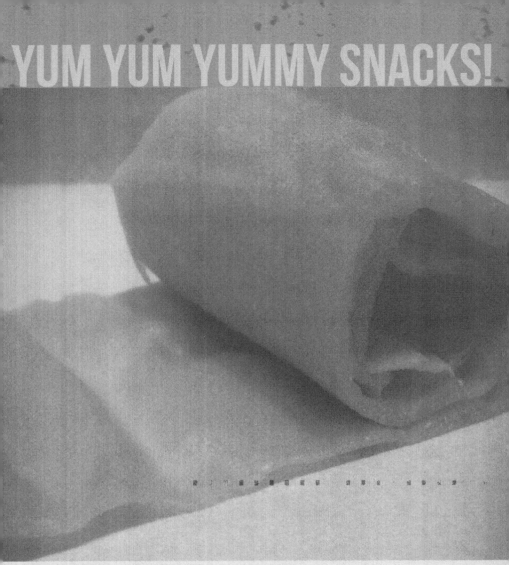

Mango-Fruit Roller

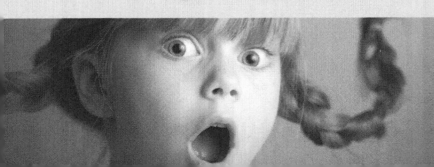

MANGO-FRUIT ROLLER

All we can say about this healthy version of a fruit rollup is... YUM! For this recipe, we thawed out frozen mango and pineapple the night before, so there was no chopping involved. You can use three cups of any fruit combination, though. Try apple with cinnamon for autumn, or maybe fresh strawberries with juicy ripe pear. The possibilities are endless.

Mango-Fruit Roller Recipe

Ingredients:

- 2 cups peeled, chopped mango (fresh or frozen, thawed)
- 1 cup chopped pineapple (fresh or frozen, thawed)
- 2 tsp raw honey (optional)

Directions: Combine all ingredients in the food processor or blender. Process on high until the mixture is smooth. Set aside.

Preheat oven to its lowest possible temperature, or 170°F, whichever is lower. Line an 11 x 17" rimmed baking pan with parchment paper.

Pour the mixture onto the parchment-lined pan and spread out with the back of a rubber spatula. This will be a very thin layer of fruit puree, and it's imperative that you get it very even and smooth.

Place the pan in the oven, and allow to "bake" (or dehydrate) for 7 – 9 hours or until the puree is completely dried out and leathery. Remove from oven and cut strips lengthwise, leaving paper on (like a commercial fruit roll). Store in airtight container up to two weeks.

To serve: Peel, and eat!

Serving size: 1 strip   Yields: 10 servings
Prep time: 10 minutes   Cook time: 7 – 9 hours
Total time: 9 hours, 10 minutes

CONVENIENT CONDIMENTS

While paleo-friendly products are becoming more common, it's still very hard to find sauces and condiments that don't contain sugars, corn syrup, added food dyes and preservatives. That's why it's important to make up some basic condiments and keep them in the refrigerator, ready to use when you need a dab of flavor or the base for a glaze or marinade. You'll find these sauces as ingredients in many of the savory snack recipes in the next section.

SAUCES

- Paleo Pesto -
- Paleo Catsup -
- Paleo Mayonnaise -

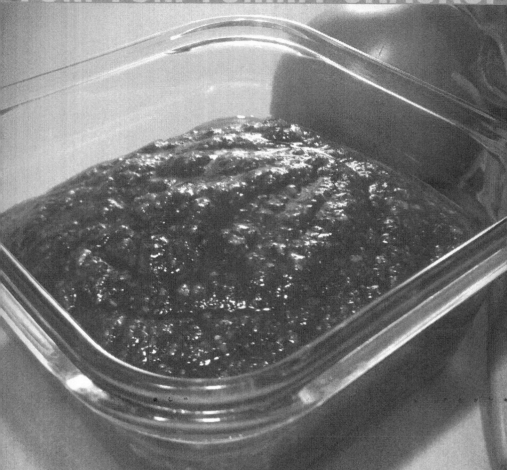

Paleo Pesto

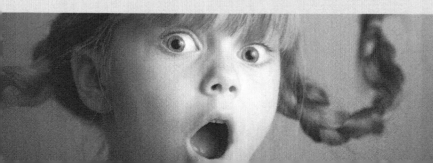

PALEO PESTO

This is a delicious substitute for traditional pesto, which generally includes Parmesan cheese. Garlic and basil are full of incredible health benefits, including antibacterial and antioxidant properties that help prevent and heal some common ailments. Incredibly versatile, you can use pesto as a spread, dip, or an ingredient in Italian-flavored dishes. You can also make variations by adding sun dried tomatoes, switching the pine nuts to walnuts or almonds, or by using spinach instead of basil for a milder flavor.

Pesto Recipe

Ingredients:

- 1 cup loosely packed fresh basil leaves
- 2 cloves garlic
- 1 cup pine nuts
- ½ cup olive oil
- Salt and pepper to taste

Directions: In a food processor or blender, pulse the pine nuts until coarsely chopped. Rinse the basil and remove stems. Place the basil leaves into your food processor or blender. Peel the garlic cloves and add them to the basil. Add olive oil, salt, and pepper. Process until the pesto has a regular consistency. It should be smooth, but not creamy. Store in an airtight glass container up to one week.

Serving size: 1 tablespoon   Yields: 40 servings
Prep time: 10 minutes   Cook time: 0
Total time: 10 minutes

YUM YUM YUMMY SNACKS!

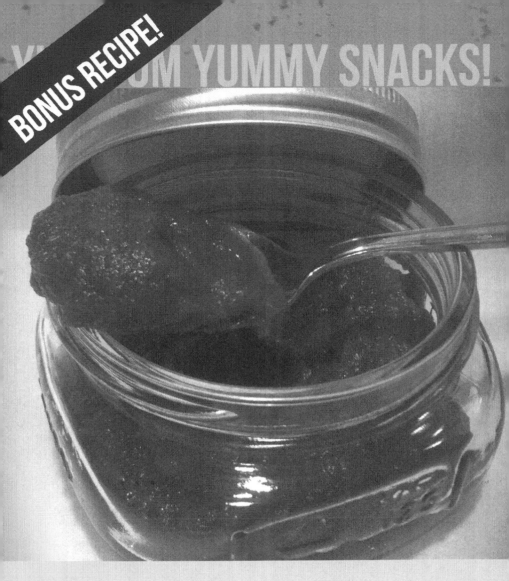

Paleo Catsup

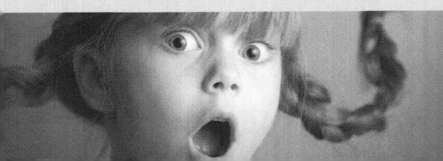

PALEO CATSUP
(BONUS RECIPE FROM *THE PALEO KID*)

Catsup isn't just a tasty condiment for French fries and beef. It's also the base for a number of different dips and sauces, like cocktail and BBQ sauces! It's best to make up a big batch of catsup and store it in a jar in the fridge. That way you can dip into it when you need it, rather than having to make it from scratch every time you want to make a sauce that uses it as a base.

Paleo Catsup Recipe

Ingredients:

* 10 oz "just prunes" organic baby food
* 10 oz tomato paste
* 3 tsp lemon juice (or unfiltered apple cider vinegar, if using)
* 3 tsp raw honey, softened
* 1/2 tsp ground mustard powder
* 1/2 tsp sea salt

Directions: In a medium sized bowl, whisk all ingredients together until smooth. Store in an airtight container in the refrigerator up to two weeks.

*This is a basic recipe. You can give it your own flare by adding garlic powder, cumin, nutmeg, cinnamon, red chili powder, and more!

Serving size: 1 tbsp   Yields: 20 servings
Prep time: 3 min   Cook time: 0
Total: 3 minutes

YUM YUM YUMMY SNACKS!

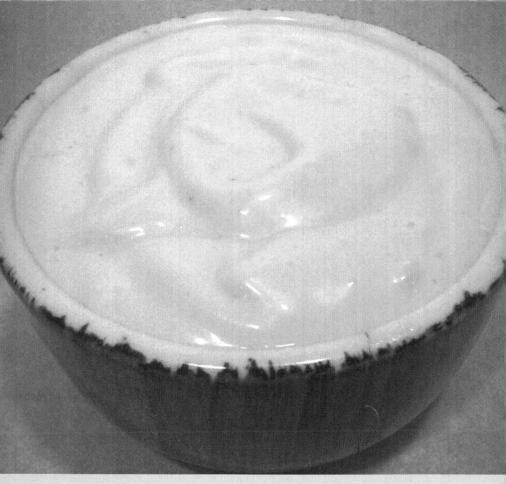

Paleo Mayonnaise

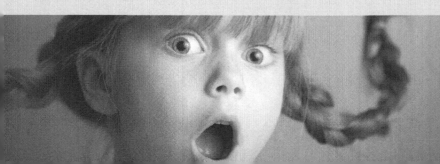

PALEO MAYONNAISE

Have you ever looked at the label on a jar of mayonnaise from the grocery store? The ingredients are definitely not in line with the Paleo diet. Containing preservatives, stabilizers, and often-artificial colors, you'll want to avoid using store bought mayo. But mayonnaise is a great spread and dip for meats, and can also transform into delicious ranch dressing, as well as spicy jalapeño dip and pesto aioli. Armed with this really simple recipe, you can enjoy all the goodness of mayo without all the junk.

Paleo Mayonnaise Recipe

Ingredients:

- 1 pastured, farm fresh egg
- 1 cup light, extra virgin olive oil or walnut oil
- 1 tbsp pure unfiltered apple cider vinegar (or substitute lemon juice if not using vinegar)
- ½ tsp sea salt
- ½ tsp dry mustard, ground
- ¼ tsp ground cayenne pepper, optional

Directions: Crack the egg into the bowl of your food processor or electric mixer. Add the vinegar, salt, mustard, and cayenne pepper and whip until frothy. Next, with the processor or mixer running, very slowly drizzle in the oil. It is crucial that you do this very slowly at first, or the oil will not integrate properly. The stream of oil should be about as wide as a thin spaghetti noodle. Keep pouring and blending until all the oil is integrated and the mixture is light and fluffy. Store in an airtight container in the refrigerator for up to one week.

*Note: Raw eggs should not be consumed by pregnant women, babies, very young children or anyone with compromised health. However, pastured eggs from local farms carry less risk of salmonella than large-scale commercially harvested eggs.

Serving size: 1 tbsp   Yields: about 20 servings
Prep time: 5 minutes   Cook time: 0
Total time: 5 minutes

NUTRITIOUS FUEL

These savory snacks fulfill our natural cravings for salt and fats that the snack-food industry would rather we fill with potato chips and crackers. Far from empty calories, these recipes can provide essential protein, fiber, and nutrients that small bodies need to fuel their high-energy lifestyle.

SAVORY SNACKS

- Egg-A Pizza -
- Deviled Eggs -
- Bacon-Wrapped Chicken Bites -
- Ham N' Onion Rollups -
- Broiled Tomatoes -
- Sausage & Pickle Sticks -
- Beef & Broccoli Bites -
- Roasted Vegetables -
- Tuna Boats -
- Turkey-Pesto Rolls -
- BBQ Chicken Cubes -
- Fresh Veggies & Ranch Dip -
- Shrimp Cocktail -

YUM YUM YUMMY SNACKS!

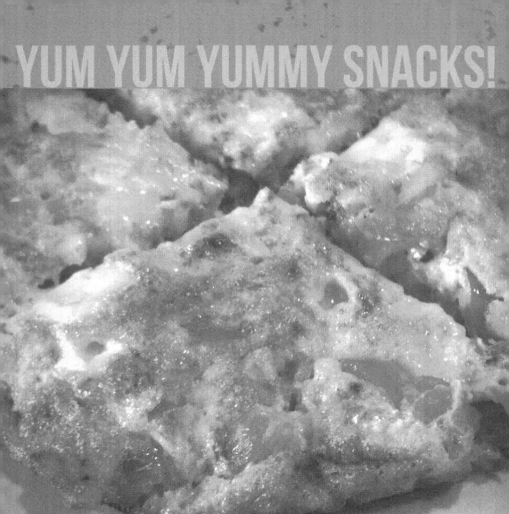

Egg-A Pizza

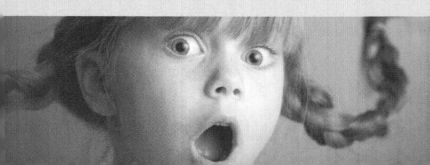

EGG-A PIZZA

Your kids will look at this snack and say, "Yay, pizza!" While it does take a bit more preparation than a simple piece of fruit, you can make it up ahead of time and store it in the fridge for a quick snack. In fact, I like to double the recipe and put some away for picnic baskets or lunch boxes. By using your kitchen staple, Paleo Pesto, you can whip up this hearty treat in no time.

Egg-A Pizza Recipe

Ingredients:

- 2 eggs
- ½ tbsp Paleo Pesto
- ¼ cup diced Roma tomato
- 1 tsp olive oil
- 1 tbsp shredded raw milk cheese (optional) * if wishing to follow an exclusively paleo diet, omit this
- Sea salt and pepper to taste

Directions: Cut the tomato in half and remove the seeds and internal membrane. Dice tomato flesh into very small pieces. Set aside.
Set a heavy bottom, oven safe six-inch omelet pan over medium heat. Evenly coat with one teaspoon of olive oil.

While the pan is heating, crack two eggs into a medium bowl. Whisk with a fork until frothy. Stir in pesto and tomato, salt and pepper. When the pan is heated, pour in the egg mixture. Turn on the timer for 2 ½ minutes. Turn on broiler to regular heat.

When the timer goes off, and the egg is done at the edges, sprinkle the cheese evenly on top of the pizza (if using). Using a hot pad or oven mitt, remove the pan from the burner and slide it under the broiler. Broil for 2 ½ to 3 minutes until the top is browned and the egg-a pizza is cooked through.

Allow the egg-a pizza to cool for at least five minutes before sliding onto a plate or cutting board. This will allow it to set completely, so it doesn't fall apart! Cut into slices and serve plain or with marinara sauce for dipping.

Serving size: ½ pizza   Yields: 2 servings
Prep time: 5 minutes   Cook time: 6 min Cool time: 5 min
Total time: 16 min

YUM YUM YUMMY SNACKS!

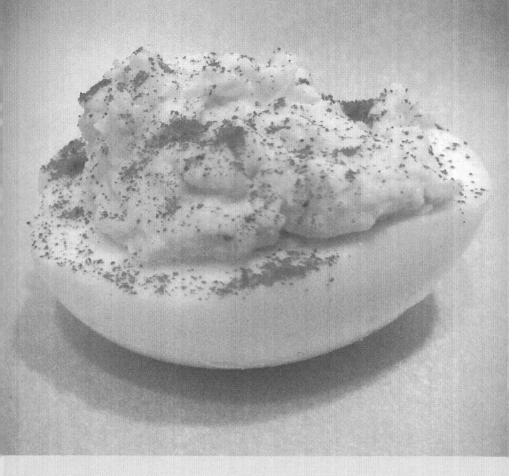

Deviled Eggs

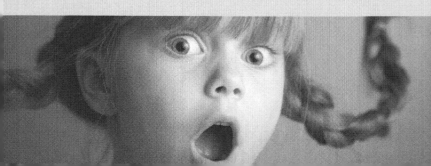

DEVILED EGGS

Eggs are a great source of protein on the paleo diet. I like to boil a dozen at the beginning of the week just to have on hand for quick snacks. But when you don't want just a plain old egg, you can create a delicious appetizer in just a few quick steps.

Deviled Eggs Recipe

Ingredients:

- 2 boiled eggs
- 3 tsp paleo mayonnaise
- Dash paprika (optional)

Directions: Slice the boiled eggs in half lengthwise. Gently remove the yolk into a medium sized bowl. To the yolk, add 3 teaspoons mayonnaise. Mash with a fork, and then whip until the mixture is smooth. Scoop about 1 teaspoon of mixture back into each egg-white half. Sprinkle with paprika.

Serving size: 2 halves Yields: 2 servings
Prep time: 5 minutes (from pre-boiled eggs) Cook time: 0
Total time: 5 minutes

YUM YUM YUMMY SNACKS!

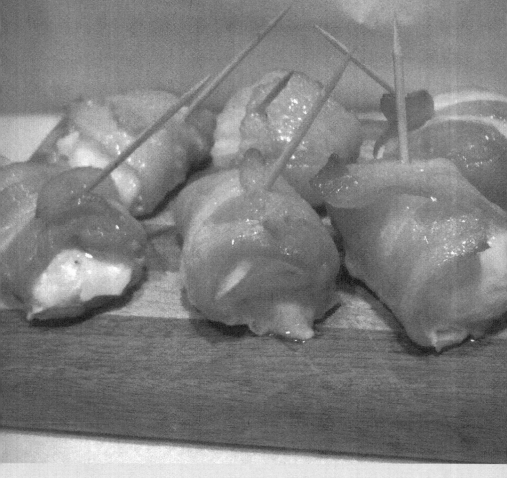

Bacon-Wrapped Chicken Bites

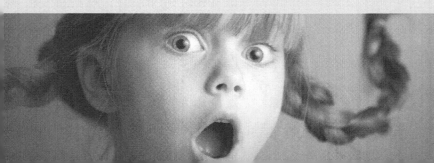

BACON-WRAPPED CHICKEN BITES

We all know that anything wrapped in bacon is going to be delicious, but these simple chicken bites are "baconlicious!" They are really easy to make, and could be accompanied by various dips if your children are big dunkers. Make a double batch and put them in the fridge for up to five days, because they're just as good reheated or cold for lunch boxes.

Bacon-Wrapped Chicken Bites Recipe

Ingredients:

- 1 medium boneless, skinless, free range organic chicken breast
- 3 strips uncured bacon

Directions: Preheat oven to 375°F. Rinse chicken breast and pat dry with paper towel. On a cutting board, slice chicken into six even chunks.

Cut strips of bacon in half cross-wise. Wrap one bacon-half around a chunk of chicken and secure with toothpick. Repeat until all the chicken and bacon are used.

Place on a rimmed baking sheet and bake for 18 – 20 minutes until the chicken is cooked through and the bacon is crisp.

Serving size: 1 breast   Yields: 6 servings
Prep time: 7 minutes   Cook time: 20 minutes
Total time: 27 minutes

YUM YUM YUMMY SNACKS!

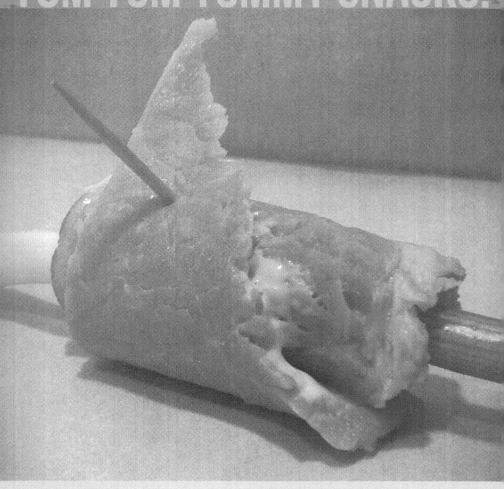

Ham'N Onion Rollups

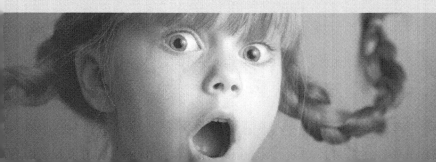

HAM N' ONION ROLLUPS

On the paleo diet, traditional sandwiches are off the menu. But with thin deli-style slices of meat, you can have all the flavors of a sandwich without the bread. The next time you bake a ham, slice a pound thin and keep it in the refrigerator for meat and veggie rollups.

Ham N' Onion Rollups Recipe

Ingredients:

- 3 slices thick-cut ham
- 3 green onions
- 3 tsp paleo mayonnaise
- 3 toothpicks

Directions: Lay the ham slices out flat on a plate. Spread each slice with one-teaspoon mayonnaise. Rinse onions and trim off root ends and dark green leafy shoots. Lay one onion on the end of each ham slice. Roll up the ham around the onion and secure with a toothpick.

Serving size: 1 roll   Yields: 3 servings
Prep time: 5 minutes   Cook time: 0
Total time: 5 minutes

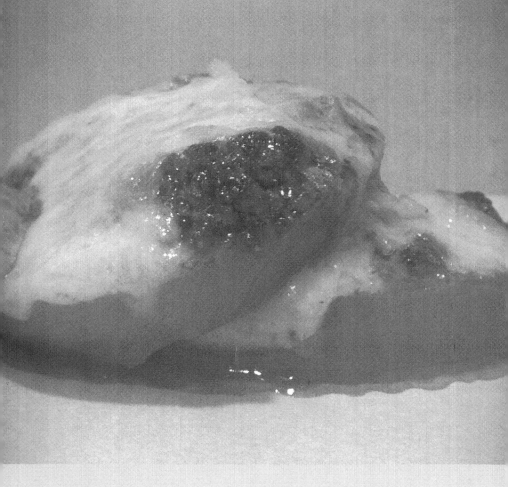

YUM YUM YUMMY SNACKS!

Broiled Tomatoes

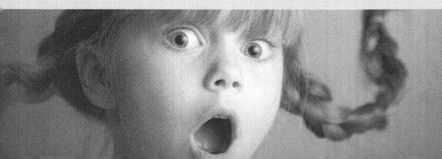

BROILED TOMATOES

With this pesto on hand, you can turn a fresh tomato into a delicious and hearty Italian-inspired snack. If you are someone who doesn't like hot tomatoes, or you don't have time for broiling, you can always just spread the pesto on the raw tomato slices and eat it cold. It's perfect, either way!

Broiled Tomato Recipe

Ingredients:

- 1 medium ripe tomato
- 4 tsp pesto
- 2 oz raw cheese (optional)

Directions: Preheat the broiler to High. Wash and slice the tomato into slices about ¼ inch thick. You want them to retain their shape when cooked a little.

Place the tomato slices on a small, rimmed baking pan. Spread each slice with 1-teaspoon pesto and top with crumbled or shredded raw cheese.
Place under the broiler for about 3 – 5 minutes until the pesto is browning and the cheese is melted. Allow to cool slightly before using a spatula to remove to a plate. Serve warm.

Serving size: 2 slices Yields: 2 servings
Prep time: 2 minutes Cook time: 5 minutes
Total time: 7 minutes

YUM YUM YUMMY SNACKS!

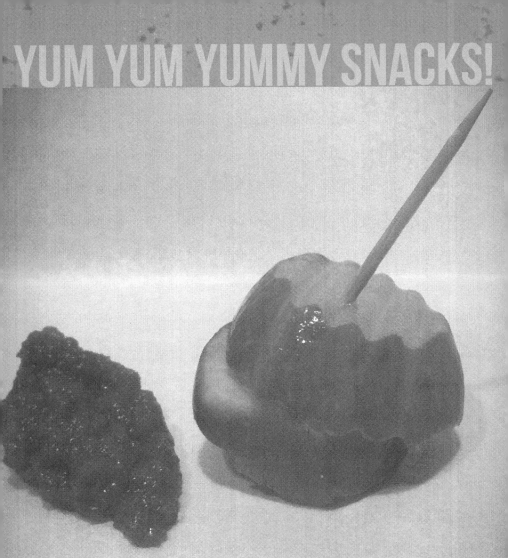

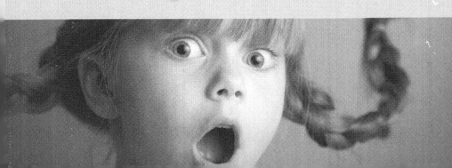

Sausage & Pickle Sticks

SAUSAGE AND PICKLE STICKS

This snack is inspired by the backyard cookout: hot dogs or smoked sausages with relish and catsup! You can get natural free-range sausages, without the nitrates and nitrites, at most health food stores and even some local grocers. I've found that another good place to get paleo-friendly meats is at our local farmer's market. If you don't have homemade pickles, just look for a natural or organic brand without any added preservatives.

Sausage And Pickle Sticks Recipe

Ingredients:

- 1 natural, precooked chicken-sausage (can substitute pork, turkey, or beef sausage)
- 9 pickle slices (home-made or natural, without added preservatives or coloring)
- 3 tsp paleo catsup
- 9 toothpicks

Directions: Slice the sausage into nine rounds. Place one pickle slice on top of each piece of sausage and spear through with a toothpick. Serve with paleo catsup.

Serving size: 3 sticks   Yields: 3 servings
Prep time: 5 minutes   Cook time: 0
Total time: 5 minutes

YUM YUM YUMMY SNACKS!

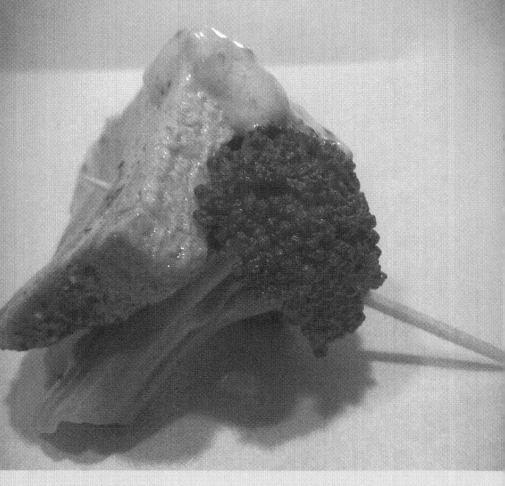

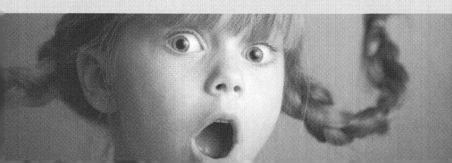

Beef & Broccoli Bites

BEEF AND BROCCOLI BITES

A thick cut of natural roast beef from the grocer's deli makes this hearty snack incredibly quick and tasty! The parboiled broccoli is tender and flavorful, complimenting the beef perfectly. Served with a quick mix of pesto and mayo, this is a winning combination for even the pickiest kid.

Beef And Broccoli Bites Recipe

Ingredients:

- 9 broccoli florets
- ¼ lb roast beef (precooked)
- 9 toothpicks
  Pesto Mayonnaise
- 1 ½ tbsp pesto
- 1 ½ tbsp paleo mayonnaise

Directions: To make the beef and broccoli: In a small saucepan, bring two cups of water to a boil. Rinse and trim the broccoli florets. When the water is boiling, drop in the broccoli. Cook for no more than one minute. Remove immediately to a colander and rinse with cold water to stop the cooking. Now your broccoli is parboiled.

With a sharp knife and cutting board, cut the roast beef into 9 squares. Stack one broccoli floret on top of each beef square, and spear through with a toothpick.

To make the dipping sauce: Mix pesto with mayonnaise until completely integrated. Serve alongside the beef and broccoli bites.

Serving size: 3 bites   Yields: 3 servings
Prep time: 10 minutes   Cook time: 1 minute
Total time: 11 minutes

YUM YUM YUMMY SNACKS!

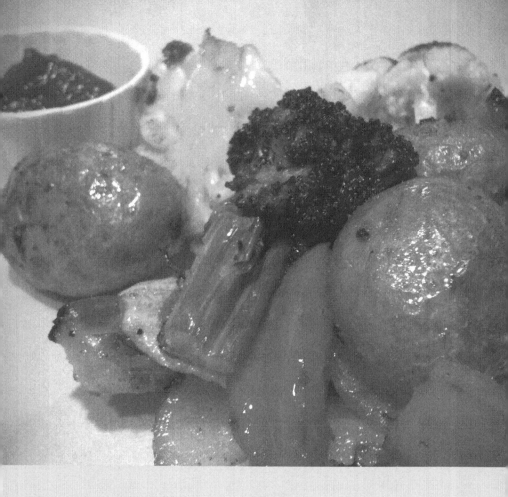

Roasted Vegetables

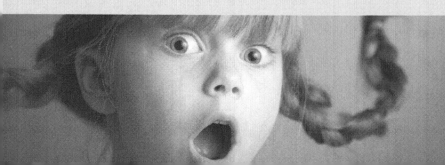

ROASTED VEGETABLES

Veggies are great raw, but roasting them often brings out flavors and textures that are surprising and delicious. Carrots and yams get sweeter, and peppers and onion caramelize for a robust, smoky flavor. If you let the roasted vegetables cool a bit before serving, little hands can pick them up and dip them into their favorite condiment.

Roasted Vegetables Recipe

Ingredients:

- 6 cups chopped mixed vegetables (I used small red potatoes, onion, red pepper, broccoli, cauliflower, and carrots)
- 3 tbsp extra virgin olive oil
- 1 tsp garlic powder
- Salt and pepper to taste

Directions: Preheat oven to 425 °F. Wash, trim, and chop the vegetables into large pieces, about 1 inch. Place the vegetables in a large bowl. Add the olive oil, garlic powder, salt and pepper. Toss to completely coat the vegetables with the oil.

Spread the vegetables out on a large rimmed baking dish. Bake for 30 – 40 minutes, turning once half way through. The vegetables should be crisp and maybe even a bit charred around the edges, and soft in the middle.

Remove from oven and serve hot with paleo catsup, BBQ sauce, or garlic mayonnaise.

Serving size: 1 cup, cooked   Yields: 4 servings
Prep time: 15 minutes   Cook time: 40 minutes
Total time: 55 minutes

YUM YUM YUMMY SNACKS!

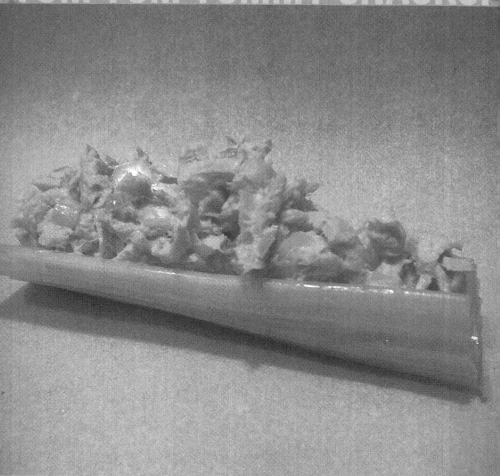

Tuna Boats

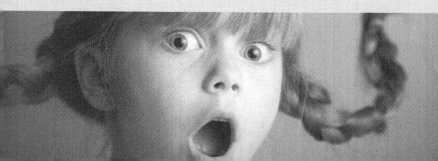

TUNA BOATS

Tuna is a heart-healthy protein, rich in the Omega-3 fatty acids known to lower bad cholesterol and raise good cholesterol levels. Combined with paleo mayo and green onion, this little celery boat bursts with so much flavor and texture; you'll think you're sitting on the wharf watching the fishing boats come in!

Tuna Boats Recipe

Ingredients:

- 1 5-oz can sustainably harvested light tuna, packed in water
- 2 tbsp Paleo mayonnaise
- 1 green onion
- 2 stalks of celery
- Sea salt and pepper to taste

Directions: Wash the celery and trim off the ends. Cut each stalk horizontally into two pieces. Set aside.

Wash, trim, and coarsely chop the green onion. Drain the water from the can of tuna and put the fish in a small bowl. Add the mayo, green onion, salt, and pepper. Smash the tuna mixture together with the back of a large fork, breaking up the larger chunks of tuna and mixing in the other ingredients. Stir and mash until the mixture takes on the consistency of a spread.

Scoop two tablespoons of the mixture onto each prepared celery-stalk half.

Serving size: 1 tuna boat   Yields: 4 servings
Prep time: 10 minutes   Cook time: 0
Total time: 10 minutes

YUM YUM YUMMY SNACKS!

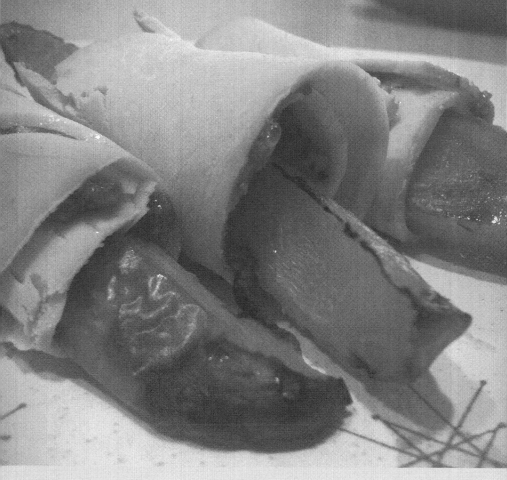

Turkey-Pesto Rolls

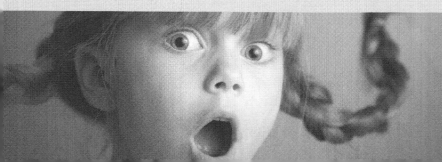

TURKEY-PESTO ROLLS

While roasting the red peppers for this recipe isn't necessary, it brings out the vegetable's sweetness and adds a smoky flavor that goes well with the turkey and pesto. You can roast the whole pepper and keep the slices in a zipper bag in the refrigerator up to four days.

Turkey-Pesto Rolls Recipe

Ingredients:

- 6 slices roasted turkey breast
- 6 slices red bell pepper (about 1/2 pepper)
- 6 tsp pesto

Directions: To roast the peppers: Turn the broiler on to high. Wash the red pepper and then quarter it lengthwise. Slice 1/2 of the pepper into six long sections. Save the rest of the pepper for later, or double the recipe! Place the pepper slices skin-side-up on a small baking tray. Broil for about 5 minutes until the skin of the pepper is charred. Remove from broiler and let sit a few minutes.

To prepare the roll: Lay the slices of turkey out on a plate or cutting board. Spread one teaspoon of pesto onto each slice of turkey. Lay a slice of pepper at the end of each turkey slice, and roll it up.

Serving size: 2 rolls   Yields: 3 servings
Prep time: 5 minutes   Broil time: 5 minutes
Total time: 10 minutes

YUM YUM YUMMY SNACKS!

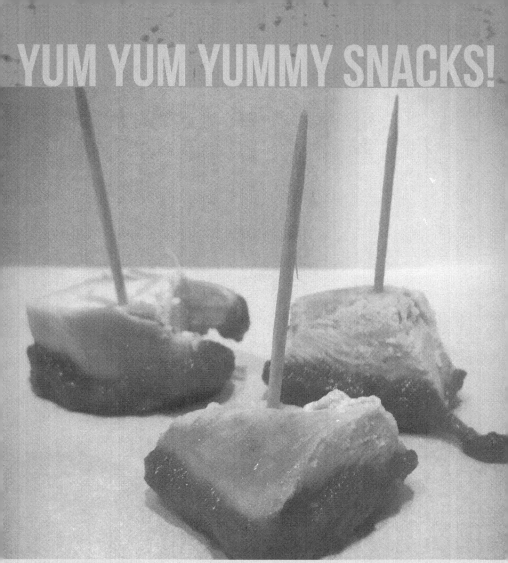

BBQ Chicken Cubes

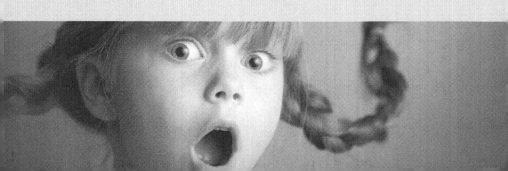

BBQ CHICKEN CUBES

This recipe is super-quick if you have an extra grilled or roasted chicken breast on hand. I always make more than needed for dinner just to have for next-day snacking, then all you have to do is cube it up and whisk up the sauce.

BBQ Chicken Cubes Recipe

Ingredients:

*   1 boneless, skinless chicken breast
*   1 tsp olive oil

Sauce:

*   1/3 c   paleo catsup
*   1/3 c   tomato sauce
*   3 tsp   pure maple syrup
*   ¼ tsp   chipotle powder
*   ½ tsp   smoked paprika
*   ½ tsp   garlic powder
*   ¼ tsp   ground cumin

Directions: If you are starting from raw chicken, the quickest way to cook it is in the frying pan. Wash and pat dry the chicken breast. Heat the olive oil in a small pan set over medium heat. Slice the chicken breast into 8 pieces. Salt and pepper to taste. Cook the chicken cubes in the pan, stirring occasionally, until the internal temperature reaches 165°F, and the juices run clear. About 7 minutes.

To make the BBQ sauce: In a medium bowl, whisk together all sauce ingredients until they reach a smooth consistency.

Spear each chicken piece with a toothpick and serve with BBQ sauce. There will be plenty of leftover sauce, which can be stored in an airtight container in the refrigerator up to one week.

Serving size: 4 pieces   Yields: 2 servings (with leftover sauce)
Prep time: 10 minutes   Cook time: 7 minutes
Total time: 17 minutes

YUM YUM YUMMY SNACKS!

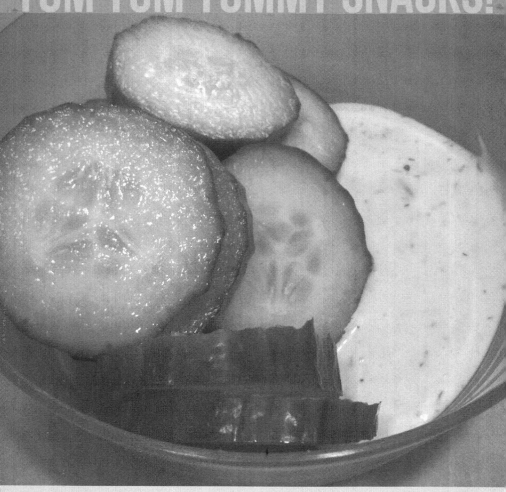

Fresh Veggies & Ranch Dip

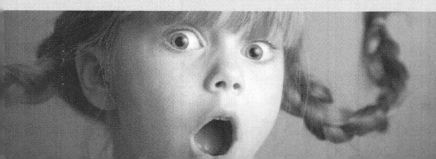

FRESH VEGGIES AND RANCH DIP

Most kids love ranch dressing. It's creamy and full of flavorful herbs that compliment any vegetable... or fruit, as in the case of cucumbers or tomatoes. With your paleo mayo already prepared and waiting the refrigerator, ranch dressing is just a few short steps away.

Fresh Veggies And Ranch Dip

Ingredients:

- 2 c   Cut fresh vegetables (I used cucumbers)

Dip:

- ½ c   Paleo mayonnaise
- 1 tsp   Chopped fresh chives
- 1/8 tsp   Each: Dried parsley, dried dill, garlic powder, onion powder
- Sea salt and black pepper to taste

Directions: Wash, peel, and cut the vegetables. Arrange on a plate or in a bowl.

For the dip: Whisk all ingredients together with a wire whisk until completely incorporated. Use immediately, or store in an airtight container in the refrigerator up to one week.

Serving size: 1 cup vegetables with ¼ cup dip   Yields: 2 servings
Prep time: 10 minutes   Cook time: 0
Total time: 10 minutes

YUM YUM YUMMY SNACKS!

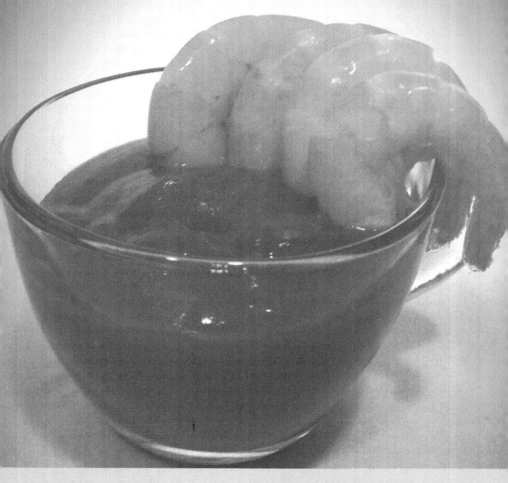

Shrimp Cocktail

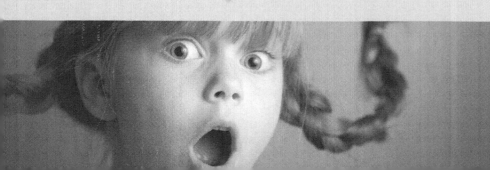

SHRIMP COCKTAIL

This cocktail sauce isn't quite as thick or sweet as the store-bought kind, but it tastes delicious with peel and eat shrimp. You can make it as zesty as you like by adding more or less hot sauce or horseradish. This is a fantastic "snack" to put out at parties, because it's loved by kids and adults alike.

Shrimp Cocktail Recipe

Ingredients:

- ½ pound large shrimp, fresh or frozen
- Sea salt for boiling

Cocktail sauce:

- ½ cup   paleo catsup
- 2 tsp   lemon juice
- 1 tsp   grated horseradish (or 2 tsp prepared)
- Dash   hot sauce, to taste

Directions: Bring two quarts of water with sea salt (to taste) to a rapid boil. Drop in shrimp and boil for 2 – 3 minutes until shrimp turns pink. Rinse immediately under cold water.

Cocktail sauce: Whisk all ingredients together until completely integrated. Pour into a serving dish and surround with shrimp. Peel, dunk, and enjoy!

Serving size: 8-10 shrimp   Yields: 2 servings
Prep time: 5 minutes   Cook time: 3 minutes
Total time: 8 minutes

A HEALTHY CHANGE

Many of us grew up on cow's milk, so the need to offer a healthy alternative to our kids without dairy (that still tastes great) can seem tricky at first when trying to make it ourselves. These two milks are a fabulous substitute to conventional milk (for children over the age of 1) and are always enjoyed by my little ones. The best part is that they are easy to make and chock full of vitamins so you can rest easy knowing that you're feeding your kids only the best.

DAIRY-FREE MILKS
- Almond Milk -
- Coconut Milk -

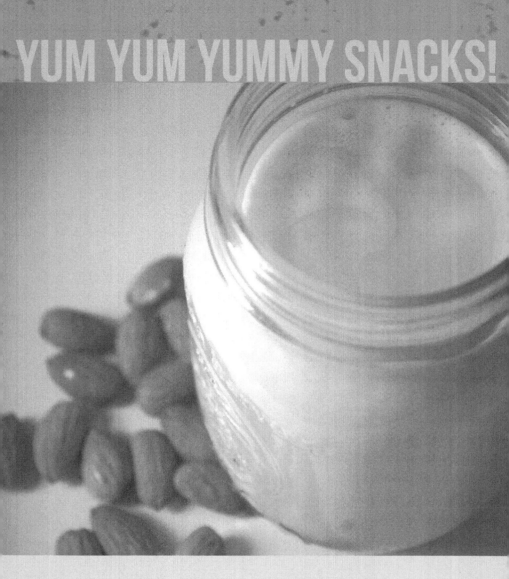

YUM YUM YUMMY SNACKS!

Almond Milk

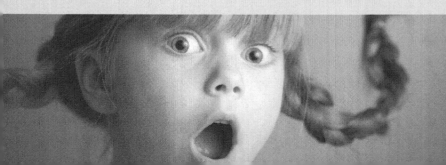

ALMOND MILK

Almond milk is one of the most nutritionally valuable milk substitutes for children. Making it yourself as opposed to buying it in the store is easy and much healthier. Your kids will love this sweet and tasty drink at any time of the day or at every meal. Almond milk is high in a number of vitamins & minerals including vitamin E, Manganese, Magnesium, Phosphorus, Potassium, Selenium, Iron, fiber, and Zinc. It is also higher in Calcium than cow's milk. It is low in calories and low in fat. Almond milk is lactose, gluten, casein and cholesterol free (and also free of saturated fats to boot). Please note that the nutritional profile for almond milk is quite different from cow's milk, breast milk, or formula. In particular, the fat content is lower than cow's milk and toddlers need extra fat in their diets so compensate accordingly (almond milk should not be used as a substitute for breast milk or formula for children under the age of 1).

Almond Milk Recipe

Ingredients:

- 1 cup raw/natural almonds
- 4 cups water
- 4 to 5 small dates
- Pinch of Celtic Sea-Salt
- ¼ to ½ teaspoon pure vanilla extract (optional)

Directions: Soak almonds and dates in water for 1 hour (ideally up to 8 hours or over night if possible). Place soaked almonds and dates in a blender or food processor. Add sea-salt and vanilla extract then blend until smooth. Pour mixture through a fine sieve, cheese cloth, or nut-milk bag and strain. Remaining pulp can be used in other recipes or baked on low in oven and ground as flour. This milk can be stored in the fridge for up to 5 days (separation will naturally occur).

To add variations to this, feel free to add raw cacao powder, almond butter, a banana, cinnamon, or mix add it into a smoothie recipe instead of cow's milk.

Serving size: 1 cup   Yields: 4 servings
Prep time: 1 hour (or up to 8)   Cook time: 0 minutes
Total time: 1 hour

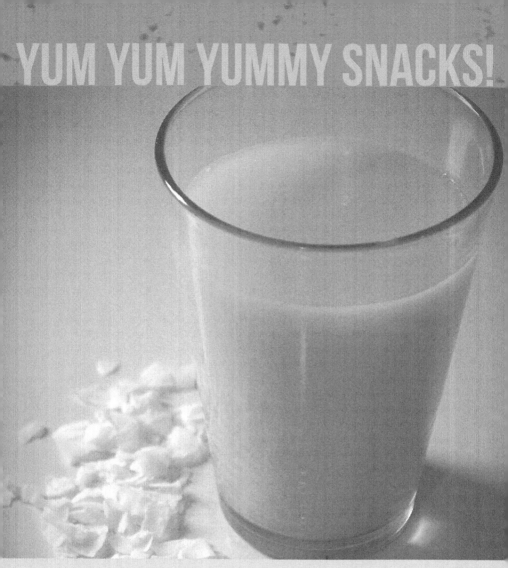

YUM YUM YUMMY SNACKS!

Coconut Milk

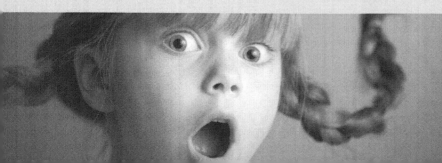

COCONUT MILK

Another excellent milk substitute is coconut milk, which is higher in Calcium than cow's milk and almond milk. Coconut milk is rich in a wide variety of minerals and vitamins such as Iron, Selenium, Sodium, Magnesium, Phosphorus, Potassium, as well as Vitamin C, E, B1, B3, B5 and B6. Coconut milk is also a good source of protein. It is believed to boost the immune system due to its fatty acids, which contain Lauric Acid. Lauric Acid has been found to be anti-viral, anti-bacterial, anti microbial and anti fungal.

Coconut Milk Recipe

Ingredients:

- ½ cup dried organic unsweetened shredded coconut (non-organic contains sulfites and tends to be sweetened)
- 4 cups very hot water
- 4 small dates (optional)
- ¼ to ½ teaspoon pure vanilla extract (optional)

Directions: If using a food processor, pulse mixture 20 times until thoroughly blended. If using a blender, blend on high for 1 to 2 minutes or until thoroughly blended. Pour mixture through a fine sieve, cheesecloth, or nut-milk bag and strain. Remaining pulp can be used in other recipes or baked on low in oven and ground as flour. This milk can be stored in the fridge for up to 5 days (separation will naturally occur).

To add variations to this, feel free to add raw cacao powder, almond butter, a banana, cinnamon, or mix add it into a smoothie recipe instead of cow's milk.

Serving size: 1 cup   Yields: 4 servings
Prep time: 10 minutes   Cook time: 0 minutes
Total time: 10 minutes

YUM YUM YUMMY PALEO!

Almond Sugar Cookies

ALMOND SUGAR COOKIES
(BONUS RECIPE FROM *THE PALEO KID*)

These are quite simply the best cookies on the planet, paleo or otherwise. Simple to make and perfectly sweet, these cookies are a versatile, filling and healthy alternative to a bakery treat. We will eat them plain as a snack, as a yummy ending to our meal, or dress them up with nut butters and fruits for lunch. When it's close to the holidays, we'll cut them into snow flake shapes and sprinkle them with a little xylitol for parties or potlucks. Shhhhh... no-one ever guesses these cookies are good for them!

Almond Sugar Cookie Recipe

Ingredients:

- 2 cups blanched almond meal
- 3 tbsp coconut oil
- 3 tbsp raw honey
- ¼ tsp baking soda*
- dash cinnamon

Directions: Preheat oven to 325°F. In a mixing bowl with an electric beater, or a food processor, combine all ingredients. Mix or process until a thick dough forms, about 3 – 5 minutes. Press dough into a soft ball and set on a sheet of parchment paper.

Place another sheet of parchment paper on top of dough ball. Roll the dough with a rolling pin to desired thickness, about ¼ inch. Cut with a round (or shaped) cookie cutter and place cut cookies on a parchment lined cookie sheet. When you've cut as many shapes as possible, press remaining scraps of dough back into a ball and re-roll. Repeat this until all the dough has been used. Generally, I use the small-sized mason jar canning ring because it cuts the perfect size for my needs.

Bake about 7 – 9 minutes until the cookies are golden brown. Let cook on the cookie sheet until cooled and set, about five minutes.

*Some paleo dieters do not use baking soda. You can omit the soda here, but your cookies will be crisp rather than soft and chewy.

Serving size: 1 cookie   Yields: 12 servings
Prep time: 15 min   Bake time: 7 – 9 min
Total: 24 min

GRAB N' SNACK

Let's face it; as much as we'd love to slow it down sometimes, we live in a fast-paced world where we don't always have time to cook. Don't worry, there are a lot of healthy snacks that you or your children can grab and eat on the run. Here's my short-list of healthy, yummy, quick foods that can be eaten straight out of the fridge or cupboard.

- Roasted, unsalted nuts
- Dried fruits
- Fresh fruits
- Fresh vegetables
- Natural, no sugar added applesauce cups
- Natural deli meats
- Boiled eggs
- Beef jerky
- Cold roasted chicken
- Raw cheese cubes (if using)
- Sweet potato chips
- Natural pre-packaged fruit leathers

ABOUT THE AUTHOR

Kate Evans Scott is a stay-at-home mom to a preschooler and a toddler. In her former life she worked in graphic design and publishing which she now draws from to create inspiring books for young children and parents.

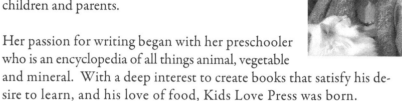

Her passion for writing began with her preschooler who is an encyclopedia of all things animal, vegetable and mineral. With a deep interest to create books that satisfy his desire to learn, and his love of food, Kids Love Press was born.

MORE BOOKS FROM KIDS LOVE PRESS:

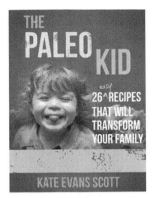

Available Now on Amazon

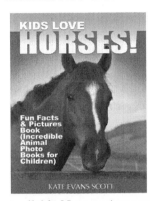

Available Now on Amazon

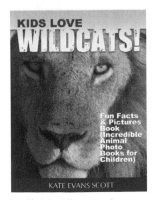

Available Now on Amazon

NOTES

Made in the USA
Lexington, KY
08 September 2013